ALL YOU WANTED TO KNOW ABOUT

Aromatherapy

Sumeet Sharma

New Dawn

NEW DAWN
An imprint of Sterling Publishers (P) Ltd.
A-59, Okhla Industrial Area, Phase-II,
New Delhi-110020.
Tel: 26387070, 26386209
Fax: 91-11-26383788: E-mail: mail@sterlingpublishers.com
ghai@nde.vsnl.net.in
www.sterlingpublishers.com

All You Wanted to Know About - Aromatherapy

ISBN 978 81 207 2272 9
Reprint 2001, 2010

Printed in India

Printed and Published by Sterling Publishers Pvt. Ltd.,
New Delhi-110 020.

Contents

Introduction

The word aromatherapy means 'treatment using scents'. It refers to the use of essential oils in Holistic Healing to improve health and emotional well being and in restoring balance to the body. Essential oils are aromatic essences extracted from plants, flowers, trees, fruit, bark, grasses and seeds. There are more than 150 types of oils that can be extracted. These oils have distinctive therapeutic, psychological and physiological properties that improve health and prevent illness. All essential oils have unique healing and valuable antiseptic properties. Some oils are anti-viral, anti-inflammatory, pain-relieving, anti-depressant, stimulating, relaxing, expectorating, support digestion and have diuretic properties too.

Essential oils get absorbed into our body and exert an influence on it. The residue gets dispersed from the body naturally. They can also affect our mind and emotions. They enter the body in three ways: by inhalation, absorption and consumption.

From the chemist's point of view, essential oils are a mixture of organic compounds viz., ketones, terpenes, esters, alcohol, aldehyde and hundreds of other molecules which are extremely difficult to classify, as they are small and complex. The essential oils' molecules are small. They penetrate human skin easily and enter the blood stream directly and finally get flushed out through our elementary system.

A concentrate of essential oils is not greasy; it is more like water in texture and evaporates quickly. Some of them are light liquid insoluble in water and evaporate instantly when exposed to air. It would take 100 kg of lavender to yield 3 kg of lavender oil; one would need 8 million jasmine flowers to yield barely 1 kg of jasmine oil.

Some of these aroma oils are very expensive. They are extracted using maceration. The purification process called defleurage is employed, and in some cases fat is used instead of oil. Then this process, called enfleurage, is used for final purification.

Some of the common essential oils used in aromatherapy for their versatile application are:

1. Clary Sage (Salvia Scarea)
2. Eucalyptus (Eucalyptus Globulus)
3. Geranium (Pelargonium Graveolens)
4. Lavender (Lavendula Vera Officinals)
5. Lemon (Citrus Limonem)
6. Peppermint (Mentha Piperita)
7. Petitgrain(Citus Aurantium Leaves)

8. Rosemary (Rosmarinus Officinals)
9. Tea-tree (Melaleuca Alternifolia)
10. Ylang Ylang (Cananga Odorata)

The oils mentioned can be good in a beginner's kit.

Origin of Aromatherapy

The oldest use of aroma oils is known to be as old as 6000 years back when Egyptian physician, Imhotep, the then God of Medicine and Healing recommended fragrant oils for bathing and massaging. In 4,500 B.C. Egyptians used myrrh and cedar wood oils for embalming their dead and 6,500 years later the preserved mummies prove the fact discovered by the modern researchers that the cedar wood contains natural fixative and strong anti-bacterial and anti-septic properties.

Hippocrates, the Greek father of Medicine, recommended regular aromatherapy baths and scented massages. This is what he effectively used to ward off plague from Athens.

Romans utilised essential oils for pleasure and to cure pain and also for their popular perfumed baths and massages. Emperor New being indulgent in orgies, feasts and fragrances employed rose frequently to cure his headaches, indigestion and to maintain his high spirits while enjoying amusements.

During the great plague in London in 1665, people burnt bundles of lavender, cedar wood and cypress in the streets and carried posies of the same plants as their only defence to combat infectious diseases.

Aromatherapy received a wider acceptance in the early twentieth century. In 1930s Rene- Maurice-Gatte Fosse, a French chemist, diped his burnt hand in lavender oil. To his surprise the wound healed very quickly without any infection or scarring. He did considerable research on various oils and their therapeutic and psychotherapeutic properties.

Dr Jean Volnet, French army surgeon extensively used essential oils in World War II. It was Madame Morquerite Murry who gave the holistic approach to aroma oils by experimenting with them for individual problems.

Today, research have proved the multiple use of aroma oils. Medical research in the recent years has uncovered the fact that the odours we smell have a significant impact on the way we feel. Smells act directly on the brain like a drug according to scientific research. For instance smelling lavender increases alpha wave frequency in the back of the head and this state is associated with relaxation.

Essential oils like spiritual healing(Reiki, Pranic, Magnified), homeopathic, herbal and flower remedies have a life force that vibrates within the body and the benefit exerted is too subtle to evaluate.

How does Aroma oils work?

Dr Alan Huch, a neurologist, psychiatrist and also the director of Smell and Taste Research Centre in Chicago says, "Smell acts directly on the brain, like a drug". Our nose has the capacity to distinguish 1,00,000 different smells, (many of which) affect us without our knowing about the same.

The aroma enters our nose and connects with cilia, the fine hair inside the nose lining. The receptors in the cilia are linked to the olfactory bulb which is at the end of the smell tract. The end of the tract is in turn connected to the brain itself. Smells are converted by cilia into electrical impulses that are transmitted to the brain through olfactory system. All the impulses reach the limbic system. Limbic system is that part of the brain which is associated with our moods, emotions, memory and learning. All the smell that reaches the limbic system has a direct chemical effect on our moods.

For example smelling lavender increases alpha waves in the brain and it is this wave that helps us to relax. A whiff of jasmine increases beta waves in the brain and this wave is associated with an increased agile and alert state.

Limbic system is also a storehouse of millions of remembered smells. That is why the mere fragrance of haystack takes us back to childhood.

The molecular sizes of the essential oils are very tiny and they can easily penetrate through the skin and get into the blood stream. It takes anything between a few seconds to two hours for the essential oils to enter the skin and within 4 hours the toxins get out of the body through urine, perspiration and excreta.

Aroma oils work like magic for stress-related problems, psychosomatic disorders, skin infections, hair loss, inflammations, pains arising from muscular or skeletal disorders to name some of the application. Actually essential oils have innumerable applications.

In Bristol, lavender oil was used on 28 patients who had undergone by-pass surgery. 24 of them reported reduced breathing rates, lower blood pressure and anxiety levels.

In Paris, in 1985, 28 women were given treatment for thrush using essential oils. After 90 days the clinical examination showed that 21 of them had been cured completely.

Essential oils are safe to use. The only caution being they should never be used directly because some oils may irritate sensitive skin or cause photo-sensitivity. They should be blended in adequate proportion with the carrier oils. A patch test is necessary to rule out any reactions.

How to use Aroma oils

Essential oils can be used in a variety of ways at home and place of work. Some of the common ways are:

Inhalation: Add 2-3 drops of essential oil depending on which oil you have selected to the hot boiling water and inhale the steam by covering your head with a towel to stop the steam from escaping. Steaming also helps open the pores of the skin and thus more oil is absorbed giving the additional benefit of a facial. The bowl which has the hot water and the aroma oil could be left under the bed so that the room is enveloped in aromatic fragrance. This could be done with the same bowl of hot steaming water and essential oil which had been used earlier for inhalation. A drop or two sprinkled on a handkerchief can give a lasting benefit of the aroma oil. For a very peaceful and relaxed sleep one or two drops of essential oils on a tissue kept inside the pillow or cushion could be used.

Diffusers and Vapourisers: Diffusers are generally made of ceramic or clay. The diffuser has a cave like opening to house small candles or earthen oil lamps and the top is shaped like a curved cup to hold a little water and few drops of aroma oil. Fill the top cup with water, add a few drops of essential oils depending on the oil chosen then light the candle or the lamp. For the oil lamp to last for a long duration, add castor oil to the earthen lamp because castor oil burns for a very long time as compared to the other oils used to light a lamp. Once the water and oil heat up, evaporation takes place and the whole atmosphere is filled with the aromatic scent. The process of evaporation continues for nearly five to six hours. This is ideal for presenting a conducive ambience during a gathering or even in bedrooms, hotels, living-rooms, etc., and anywhere where scented air is required. One can get instant relief from pain, a relaxed and positive feeling prevails when the right oil is used. One needs to be careful in choosing the right essential oil.

Vaporisers are the insect repellents used normally in the form of mats or other types of vaporisers kept for repelling insects. One could reuse the used mats by adding 2-3 drops of essential oil of your own choice and keeping them lit (electrically). Slowly the smell will get released and the area would be filled with soothing aroma. Lemon or rosemary are beneficial for offices, lavender for bedroom, antiseptic tea-tree for disinfecting a sick room and citronella for repelling the insects.

Massage: The most common form of treatment is massage because the dual benefits of touch therapy and scent therapy are simultaneously enjoyed. Massage improves the circulation of the blood, tones the muscles, detoxify toxins, releases trapped energy from tense muscles. The fragrance triggers a sense of pleasure and well being. The penetration of essential oil through the skin during massages is high. Generally carrier oils like sunflower, coconut, olive, sweet almond, sesame and vegetable oils are mixed with aroma oils. The aroma oils should not be used for massages directly without dilution. About 10 drops or 1 teaspoon of essential oil can be mixed to about 30 ml of carrier oil. This makes a very rejuvenating massage oil.

Baths: This is an easy way to relax using essential oils. Add the selected oil to your bathtub, stir the water well and spend 20 minutes in the tub. The aroma oil enters the body through the skin to give lasting benefits. Just a few drops are required to be added to the bathtub. The essential oils can also be added to a bucket of water instead of a bathtub. Mix the oil in the water properly, as some of the aroma oils are insoluble in water.

Foot Bath: You can immerse your feet in a bowl of luke warm water to which 2-3 drops of essential oil is added. This is a very refreshing experience after a hard days work and if you have sweaty and smelly feet then too this foot bath is very profitable.

Pot Pourri: Pot Pourri as the name suggests is a mixture of dried flowers, herbs, grass and seed pods. Few drops of essential oil added to the pot pourri and kept in a bowl would keep giving out aromatic fragrance for 4-6 weeks.Another more effective method would be to keep the pot pourri mixture after adding the essential oil in a closed container overnight so that the oil gets absorbed. The following morning the box can be kept open and the lingering aroma would fill the area.

Bed Time: Sprinkle 2-3 drops on the pillow cover or on a tissue that can be placed under the pillow or cushion cover and inhaled just before sleeping or while sleeping. This can be very useful in treating headaches, stress, tension and in boosting confidence. Some of the essential oils act as an aphrodisiac too.

Compresses: Both cold and hot compresses are profitable. Add 2-3 drops of aroma oil to a bowl of hot (depending on how much of heat you can withstand) or warm water and dip a hand towel or piece of cotton to enable it to absorb the mixture then squeeze out the excess water and place the towel or cotton on the area to be treated. Leaving the compress on the area for 2 hours is quite beneficial. Oil like lavender is usually used. This provides relief when used over bruises, skin problems and pre menstrual syndromes. To make cold compress, add 6 cubes of ice to a bowl with 2-3 drops of essential oil and dip a hand towel or a piece of cotton to absorb the mixture then squeeze out the excess water and place the towel or cotton on the area to be treated. Cold compress is highly helpful in treating burns, sore feet, hangover, sprains and headaches. After a facial the use of hot and cold compress alternately helps the skin.

Oral Intake: It is an accepted practice abroad to take essential oil orally as it is safe. However, care should be taken to take it only under the supervision or guidance of an experienced aromatherapy practitioner. Few oils can be taken internally in prescribed dosage for a particular problem like indigestion under the guidance of a qualified therapist only.

Beauty Treatment: Aroma oils have been used as an application for the skin from times immemorial. As they are highly soothing in treating and enhancing the natural beauty of the skin they can be safely incorporated in facials, massages, manicures, pedicures, scalp treatment, hair wash, hair treatment along with other creams and oils. Rose, chamomile, lemon, lavender, geranium, sandalwood are some good oils for facials irrespective of the fact that beauty treatment is given to normal, mature, dry, oily, sensitive or problem skin. Either one of these or a combination of two of them could be used. The carrier oils that are helpful in a beauty treatment are sweet almond, wheat germ, peach kernel, apricot kernel and sunflower. Steam facials with essential oils are also rejuvenating and help in improving the skin texture.

Room Sprays: There is a call for protecting the environment and this is becoming a prime concern worldwide. Aerosols are being discouraged due to their ozone depleting properties. Essential oils are natural and hence they could be used liberally to deodorise a room, freshen and scent your bathroom, living-room, bedroom, dining-room, office cabin, etc. Merely add 10-12 drops of aroma oil to half a litre of water and spray the mixture with the help of a spray bottle. Oils like lavender, lemon, peppermint, pine and rosemary are best for this application. Cupboards, wardrobes can also be disinfected. If a room smells of dampness or there are moulds in the hotel rooms, houses, offices or factories and shops the essential oil along with water can be sprayed.

Insect Repellents: Essential oils are excellent fragrant dispenser and non toxic insecticides. Just 2-3 drops of essential oil can be used on pillow covers, mattresses or used mosquito mats (this can be electrically reused) or applied to the exposed skin after blending with carrier oil before going to bed to repel insects. Lemongrass is best for flying insects, tea-tree for ants and fleas, thyme for crawling pests, camphor for moths and citronella for mosquitoes. Even delicate plants(both indoor and outdoor) can be protected from insects by spraying the above essential oils to the roots of the plant.

Miscellaneous Uses: Aroma oil can be added to the water used for cleaning the house. It can be used to wipe the kitchen counter, platform, dining tables, babies' nappies for disinfecting purpose and also to wash the baths and toilets.

Aroma oils have versatile applications and innumerable benefits and can be made a part of our daily routine.

Essential oils and their benefits

Amrette Seed

Botanical name: Abelmoschus Moschatus

Plant part: Seeds

Properties: Warmth-giving, relaxing, stimulating, calming

Quantity: 2-3 drops

Application: Helpful in relieving anxiety, fatigue, depression or other stress-related conditions, muscular aches, pains, cramps and poor circulation. Is an aphrodisiac. Excellent to freshen up tired and hurting feet.

Precaution: Use in low dosage. Avoid very frequent massages or baths.

Aniseed

Botanical name: Pimpenella Anisum

Plant part: Seed pod

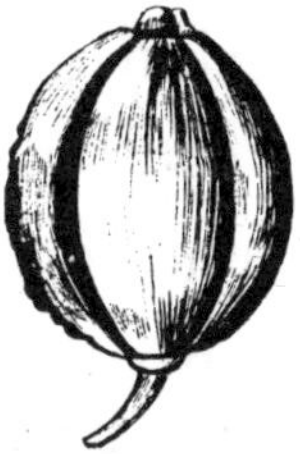

Properties: Warming, stimulating

Quantity: 3-5 drops

Application: Digestive stimulant. Helpful in treating coughs, bronchitis and catarrh.

Angelica

Botanical name: Angelica Archangelica

Plant part: Root, seed, fruit

Properties: Expectorant, digestive stimulant, relaxing

Quantity: 2-3 drops

Application: Useful for colds, coughs, flu, muscular pains and aches, rheumatism. Helps in digestion. Also useful in healing smoker's cough.

Precaution: Avoid during pregnancy. Can cause photosensitivity so avoid exposure to sun after use.

Basil

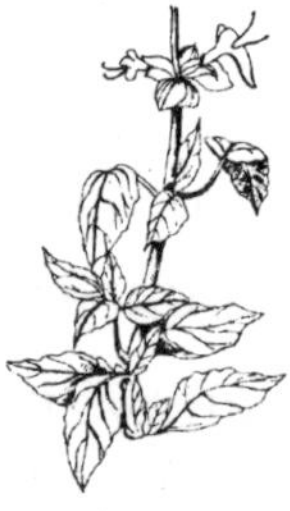

Botanical name: Ocimum Basilicum

Part of Plant: Leaves

Properties: Uplifting, refreshing

Quantity: 2-3 drops

Application: Good for students and executives. Helps in relieving nervous tension, stress, mild anxiety, nausea, indigestion, flatulence, loss of appetite, temporarily relieves cough, sinusitis, flatulence, cold, fever, bronchitis, earaches, eases muscular pains, spasm, rheumatic and arthritic pains. It also acts as an insect repellent

Precaution: Avoid during pregnancy.

Bergamot

Botanical name: Citrus Aurantium

Part of Plant: Peel of the fruit

Properties: Calming, refreshing, rejuvenating

Quantity: 3-5 drops

Application: Heals wounds and relieves ulcers, treats eczema, psoriasis (stress related) and PMT(Pre Menstrual Tension). Works as an appetiser. Beneficial in treating oily skin problems. Relieves respiratory infections viz bronchitis, sore throat and tonsilitis, colic, flatulence and indigestion. Beneficial in treating anxiety, depression, mental and psychological disturbances. Acts as an antiseptic for urinary tract problem, cystitis. Effective in treating cold sores, chicken pox and shingles.

Precaution: Avoid using on sensitive skin as it can cause irritation. Avoid exposure to sun as it can increase skin's photosensitivity

Black Pepper

Botanical name: Piper Nigrum

Plant Part: Berry

Properties: Warming, strenthening

Quantity: 2-3 drops

Application: Helps in relieving muscular aches, pains, stiffness, fatigue. Useful in relieving physical and emotional problems. Gives temporary relief from arthritis, fibrosis, cold, flu, indigestion, respiratory infections, chills, catarrh. Helps in curing colic,flatulence, indigestion, heartburn and loss of appetite. Helps to maintain peripheral circulation, eases chilblains and tones muscles. Increases concentration and alertness.

Precaution: Use in moderation.

Camphor

Botanical name: Cinnamomum Camphora

Plant part: Wood

Properties: Relieving

Quantity: 2-3 drops

Application: Helps in treating coughs, colds, fevers, rheumatism, arthritis constipation, insomnia, sprains, depression, acne and inflammed skin.

Precaution: Use in moderation.

Cardamom

Botanical name: Elettaria cardomumum

Plant part: Seeds

Properties: Warming

Quantity: 2-3 drops

Application: Helps in relieving nausea, coughs, headaches, aches, digestion and it is a tonic.

Precaution: Use in moderation.

Chamomile

Botanical name: Matricaria Chamomilia

Plant part: Flowers

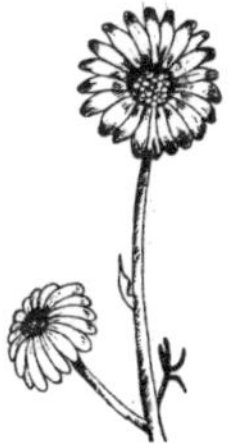

Properties: Soothes

Quantity: 3-5 drops

Application: Eases anxiety, anger and fear, helpful in treating insomnia, used for colitis, gastritis, diarrhoea, urinary tract infection, menopause and menstrual related problems. Relieves stress, depression and irritability related to PMT. Helps to relieve muscular pains, inflammation of arthritic joints and swollen joints. It is used in treating skin problems viz. psoriasis, dermatitis and eczema. Mild on children facing teething problem and earache. Soothes burns, blisters, inflammed wounds, broken capillaries. It can be used to lighten fair hair.

Precaution: Avoid during pregnancy.

Clove Bud

Botanical name: Syzygium Aromaticum

Plant part: Buds

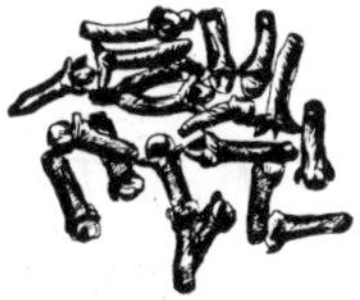

Properties: Warming and soothing

Quantity: 1-2 drops

Application: Relieves aches and pains (joints). Rheumatoid sprains, asthma, colds, flu, colic, dyspepsia, nausea, diarrhoea, toothache, ulcers, wounds, bronchitis, nervous tension, depression and stress. It is used as an effective antiseptic, and analgesic anti-bacterial. Useful as mosquito repellent and in fighting acne. Helps relieve athlete's foot and cuts.

Precaution: Use in low moderation. Avoid during pregnancy.

Cedar wood

Botanical name: Cedrus Deodora

Plant part: Wood shaving, sawdust

Properties: Sedating and relaxing

Quantity: 5-7 drops

Application: Helps relieve stress, tension, mild anxiety, arthritis, rheumatism, itching and dandruff. Symptoms of acne, pimple, oily skin, inflamed skin, eczema and blemishes can be temporarily relieved. Aids in clearing catarrh, congestion and sinusitis. Useful as insect repellent too.

Precaution: Avoid during pregnancy.

Cypress

Botanical name: Cupressus Sempervirens

Plant part: Needles, twigs

Properties: Refreshing, calming and strengthening

Quantity: 2 drops

Application: An astringent to circulation, haemorhoids, varicose veins, cellulite; brings down external bleeding and excessive perspiration and heavy menstrual flow; useful in asthma, bronchitis, dry cough, cold and flu. Helps to heal swollen breasts.

Precaution: Avoid during pregnancy.

Clary Sage

Botanical name: Salvia Sclarea

Plant part: Flowering tops

Properties: Euphoric, sensual, warming and relaxing

Quantity: 2-5 drops

Application: Useful in dealing with anxiety, stress, tension and migraine, menstrual cramps and pains, PMT, muscular tension, excessive perspiration. Being warming and relaxing nourishes conversation. Brings down high blood pressure and excessive sebum. Reduces post natal depression and eases child birth by encouraging labour. Immune system gets strengthened. Eases asthma.

Precaution: Can cause drowsiness, avoid when under alcoholic effect. Avoid during pregnancy and also if one suffers from epilepsy.

Eucalyptus

Botanical name: Eucalptus Globulus

Plant part: Leaves, twigs

Properties: Cooling and clearing

Quantity: 2-3 drops

Application: Clears stuffed nose and head. Acts as a decongestant; cures fever, cold. Relieves stress, fatigue, muscular pains, sprains, aches, rheumatism, headaches, sinusitis and mild respiratory infections. It is anti-inflammatory. Quite useful in treating wounds, burns, boils, abscesses, blisters, cold sore, shingles, blemishes, insect bites, anti-bacterial and is an insect repellent too.

Precaution: Can irritate skin. Keep away from children.

Fennel

Botanical name: Foeniculum Vulgare

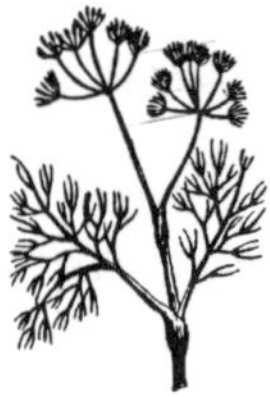

Plant part: Seeds

Properties: Calming

Quantity: 2-3 drops

Application: Useful in easing colic, constipation and digestion problems, fluid retention, cellulite, menstrual pain, PMT, menopause, nausea, flatulence and loss of appetite. Helps in fighting hangovers, increases flow of breast milk and relieves bronchitis. Cures kidney stones and relieves intestinal spasm. Has a mild diuretic and laxative effect.

Precaution: Avoid during pregnancy.

Frankincense

Botanical name: Olibanum Boswellia Carterii

Plant part: Gum resin

Property: Fortifying, soothing

Quantity: 3-5 drops

Application: Helps in meditation; slows and deepens breathing. Fortifies emotionally against nightmares, fear and grief. Balances and opens Crown chakra. It helps in healing ulcers and infected wounds. Treats dry, wrinkled, inflamed skin. It also cures coughs, laryngitis, asthma, catarrh and bronchitis. It reduces scar and promotes healing. Aids in maintaining supple skin by toning it.

Geranium

Botanical name: Pelargonium Graveolens

Plant part: Leaves, stalk, flower

Properties: Calming, balancing, relaxing, refreshing

Quantity: 5-7 drops

Application: Helps to deal with nervous tension, anxiety, mocd swings, depression, menopause problems, hot flushes, post natal depression, PMT, irregular menstruation. Treats swollen and painful breasts, fluid retention problems, emotional outbursts, irritability, throat infections. It cures colds, flu, neuralgia, sciatica, acne, bruises, burns, cuts, dermatitis, eczema, mature skin and mouth ulcers. Normalises skin imbalances. Works as insect repellant, harmonises and calms. It also acts as an astringent and cleanser.

Ginger

Botanical name: Zingiber Officinale

Plant part: Root

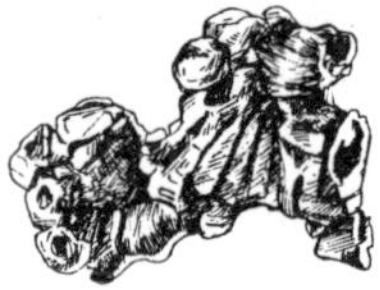

Properties: Warming, stimulating

Quantity: 2 drops

Application: Relieves colic, cramp, flatulence, nausea, travel sickness and indigestion. Cures migraine, coughs, congestion, common cold, catarrh, influenza, sore throat, sinusitis, arthritic pains, rheumatism, muscular aches, sprains and strains. Helps in blood circulation and aids memory. Heals bones and brings down temperature in fever also. Relieves morning sickness (if inhaled) in pregnancy and hangovers. Stimulates circulation, relaxes blood vessels and can also help ease angina

Precaution: May irritate sensitive skin. Use in moderation

Juniper Berry

Botanical name: Juniperus Communis

Plant part: Berries

Properties: Uplifting, refreshing, relaxing.

Quantity: 2-3 drops

Application: Used to relieve stress, anxiety, pains of joints and rheumatic pain. Heals bruises, cramps, acne, colic, coughs, arthritis, menstrual pain, less menstrual flow, swollen and painful breasts (pre-menstrual). Deals with fluid retention, cellulite, obesity, poor circulation, haemorrohoids, loss of appetite. Tones the skin

Precaution: Avoid during pregnancy and if suffering from high blood pressure. Can irritate the kidneys if used in excess.

Lavender

Botanical name: Lavandula Angustifolia

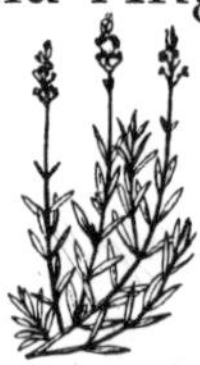

Plant part: Flowers

Quantity: 5-10 drops

Properties: Harmonising, soothing, balancing, refreshing, relaxing, calming

Application: Aids in relieving irritability (in adults and children as well), anxiety, stress. Relieves muscular aches and pains, bites and stings. Cures colds, flu, insomnia, headache, minor burns and scalds. It is anti-fungal and anti-bacterial so it is very useful in treating wounds. It can be used directly to relieve pain of minor burns and scalds. It balances and harmonises the body.

Precaution: Avoid during early pregnancy

Lemon

Botanical name: Citrus Limon

Plant part: peel of fruit

Properties: Rejuvenating, enlivening, cooling, uplifting

Quantity: 3-6 drops

Application: Helps in healing bronchial problems, colds, flu, fever, sore throat, mouth ulcers, hormonal headaches, poor circulation, high blood pressure, wounds, stress, nervous tension and counteracts acidity, Aids in clearing freckels and to rid warts. Useful for students and executives. Helps in stopping hot flushes in menopause. It has an enliving and refreshing aroma and is an effective insect repellent too.

Precaution: Causes photo-sensitivity on sensitive skin. Avoid using when going out in sun as it may irritate sensitive skin.

Lemongrass

Botanical name: Cymbogen Citratus

Plant part: Grass

Properties: Tranquilizing, soothing calming, refreshing

Quantity: 1-3 drops

Application: Helps in relieving shock, grief, trauma, depression and stress. Helps to fight lethargy, irritability during PMT and menopause, insomnia, excitability in children, chronic diarrhoea triggered due to emotional reasons. Improves skin elasticity, thread veins, stretch marks and scars. It gives relief from headaches, sore throat and mild respiratory problems. Helps in opening the skin pores, treating oily skin, curing acne and relieves indigestion.

Precaution: Avoid during pregnancy. It can also irritate skin.

Marjoram

Botanical name: Origanum Marjorana

Plant part: Flowers, leaves

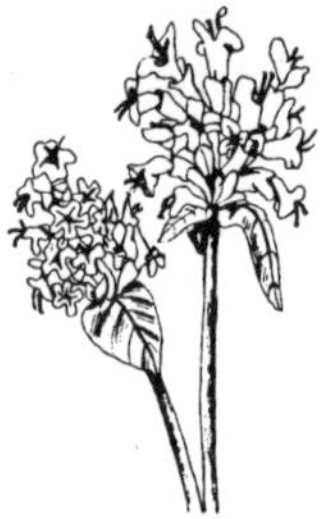

Properties: Calming, warming

Quantity: 3-5 drops

Application: Relieves anxiety, stress, high blood pressure, arthritis, rheumatism, swollen joints, asthma, colds, flu, sinusitis. Cures migraines, stomach and menstrual cramps, indigestion, constipation and flatulence. Calming to the nervous system. Reduces sexual urges, heals bruises.

Precaution: Use in moderation. Avoid during pregnancy.

Neroli

Botanical name: Citus Aurantium

Plant part: Petals

Properties: Calming, soothing, refreshing

Quantity: 1-3 drops

Application: Relieves mental lethargy, headaches, irritability caused due to menopause and PMT. It cures chronic diarrhoea due to emotional state and thread veins. Cures dryness, improves elasticity, sensitivity of skin and is also kind on mature skin. Calms excitable and restless children when used in baths before going to bed. Helps during shocks, trauma, grief and stress. Highly calming to those suffering from anxiety and fears. Helps lighten stretch marks and scars. Soothes palpitation, stress related problems and depression. Helps during pregnancy and labour.

Orange (Sweet)

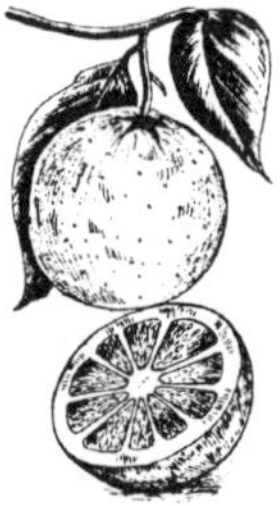

Botanical name: Citrus Aurantium

Plant part: Peel

Properties: Calming, refreshing

Quantity: 2-3 drops

Application: Effective in healing mouth ulcers, treats nervous tension, stress and anxiety. Gives relief from bronchial coughs, colds, flu and insomnia. Eases constipation and diarrhoea. It is very gentle on children brings down the fever.

Precaution: May increase skin photo-sensitivity. Avoid use before going out in the sun.

Palmarosa

Botanical name: Cymbopogon Martinii

Plant part: Grass

Properties: Clarifying, uplifting calming, refreshing

Quantity: 4-5 drops

Application: Stimulates cell regeneration, circulation, appetite. It maintains a supple skin, removes scars, helpful in treating acne, dermatitis balances sebum production, relieves indigestion, colds, flu, viruses and reduces fever.

Peppermint

Botanical name: Mentha Piperita

Plant part: Leaves

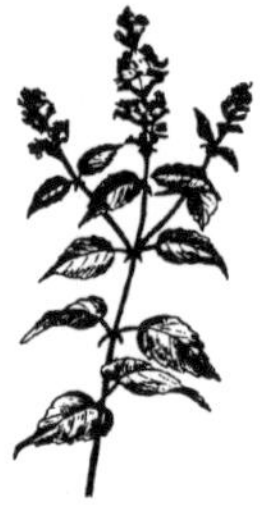

Properties: Cooling, invigorating comforting, refreshing, calming

Quantity: 1-3 drops

Application: A decongestant which gives relief from asthma, colds, flu, fever, headaches, toothaches, sinusitis, nausea, travel sickness, stomach upsets and indigestion, hangover. Cools skin inflammation, burns and sunburns as it is very refreshing skin oil. Repels mosquitoes, mice and rats.

Precaution: Avoid during early pregnancy. Use in moderation as it can irritate sensitive skin

Patchouli

Botanical name: Pogostemon Cabin

Plant part: Leaves

Properties: Exotic, calming, relaxing, enlivening, warming

Quantity: 2-4 drops

Application: Exotic aroma often used in perfumery. Emotionally enlivening, excites the senses. Helps in relieving anxiety, stress and, depression. Helps to heal chapped rough skin, wounds and sores. Being anti-inflammatory it helps cool inflammed skin. Effective in treating dandruff, scars. It is an anti-septic, astringent, anti-bacterial and insect repellent.

Precaution: Use in moderation as excess dose can cause sedation.

Petitgrain

Botanical name: Citrus Aurantium var Amara

Plant part: Leaves

Properties: Clarifying, soothing, uplifting

Quantity: 4-5 drops

Application: Useful to relieve mental strain, restlessness, anxiety, tension, stress, flatulence, dyspepsia and constipation. Helps in stimulting digestion and poor memory. Brings down acne. Reduces excessive perspiration, treats greasy skin and hair. Helps to build up resistance to illness.

Pine

Botanical name: Pinus Sylvestris

Plant part: Needles

Properties: Invigorating, refreshing

Quantity: 1-3 drops

Application: Relieves muscular aches, pains, Arthritis, rheumatism, poor circulation, asthma, bronchitis, coughs, catarrh, sinusitis, sore throats, colds, flu, nervous exhaustion, stress, fatigue, neuralgia, sciatica, poor concentration. Heals cuts and abrasions, excessive perspiration. It is also an effective insect repellent.

Rose

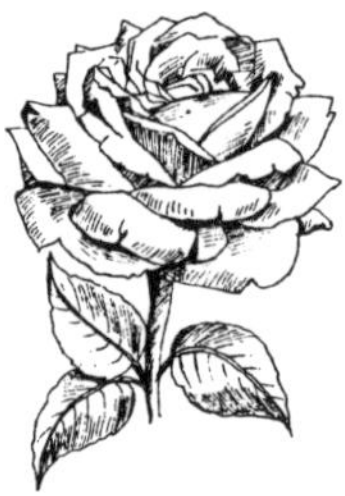

Botanical name: Rose Centifoda damascena

Plant part: Flowers and leaves

Properties: Exciting, balancing

Quantity: 1-4 drops

Application: Helps to ease depression, frigidity, nervous tension, headache and insomnia. Relieves asthma, shock, palpitations, poor circulation, dry coughs, nausea. Treats PMT, irregular or heavy menstruation, menstrual pain, impotence, irritability. Hormonally balancing. Useful also for dry, chapped, aging skin and eczema.

Rosemary

Botanical name: Rosemarinus officinalis

Plant part: Flowers, leaves

Properties: Reviving, invigorating, focusing, refreshing

Quantity: 2-4 drops

Application: Useful tonic for hair as it keeps dandruff at bay, clears lice, adds lustre to the hair. Useful in relieving stress, mental fatigue, anxiety, muscular aches and pains, rheumatism, arthritis, gout, sinusitis, migraine colds, flu, asthma, respiratory problem, poor circulation, fluid retention, cellulite, menstrual cramps, scanty flow during menstruation. Helps aid better concentration and clarity while studying.

Precaution: Avoid during pregnancy, if suffering from blood pressure or epilepsy.

Sandalwood

Botanical name: Santalum Album

Plant part: Wood

Properties: Strengthening, sedating, calming, relaxing

Quantity: 2-5 drops

Application: Helps to relieve nervous tension, depression, stress, anxiety, irritability, insomnia, dry coughs, sore throat, bronchitis, nausea, travel sickness. Heals inflamed, cracked, dry, chapped, mature, aging skin, acne, blemishes and scars. Acts as a deodoriser in case of excessive perspiration. Excites the senses. It is an effective insect repellent.

Tarragon

Botanical name: Artemisia Dracunculus

Plant part: Leaves

Properties: Calming

Quantity: 2-3 drops

Application: Useful in relieving stomach disorders, nervousness leading to butterflies or knots in the stomach, indigestion, flatulence, PMT, cramps, constipation. It is anti-spasmodic, antiseptic and slightly diruretic

Precaution: Avoid during pregnancy. Use in moderation.

Tea tree

Botanical name: Melaleuca Alternifolia

Plant part: Leaves, twigs

Properties: Soothing

Quantity: 2-5 drops

Application: Helpful in healing fungal and yeast infections, colds, influenza, cold sores, warts, burns, shock, bacterial and viral infections, stings, herpes, nappy rash and hysteria.

Thyme(White)

Botanical name: Thymus Vulgaris

Plant part: Leaves, flowers

Properties: Stimulating, invigorating

Quantity: 2 drops

Application: Helpful in relieving tension, fatigue, anxiety, headaches, skin irritations, coughs, colds, rheumatic aches and pains. Useful insect repellent. It is a very good stimulant and expectorant.

Precaution: Avoid during pregnancy. Use in moderation.

Vetiver

Botanical name: Vetiveria Zizanoides

Plant part: Roots

Properties: Balancing, calming, grounding

Quantity: 1-3 drops

Application: Helpful in relieving nervous tension, stress, muscular aches, pains, sprains, stiffness, arthritis,rheumatism, palpitation, congestion. Heals acne, blemishes, cuts and wound.

Ylang Ylang

Botanical name: Cananga Odorata

Plant part: Flowers

Properties: Balancing, relaxing

Quantity: 2-3 drops

Application: Helps to relieve tension, uncontrolled anger, stress, anxiety, rapid heart rate, rapid breathing Useful in high blood pressure, menopause, PMT, insomnia, impotence, frigidity, scalp conditioner. Useful for skin care.

Precaution: Avoid using after consuming alcohol or before driving. Use in moderation. It may cause headache and nausea when taken in excess.

How to select aroma oils

It is a fact that we get automatically attracted to pleasant smell and drift away from unpleasant smells. Subconsciously we react to smells that fall in the range of these two extreme categories. The fragrance of freshly prepared food activates the saliva when one is hungry and newly cut grass relaxes a person who is highly stressed. Aormatherapy is based on this instinctive response to smell.

An alarm clock could be preset to release a particular scent you wish to wake up to. Patients could be made to relax by inhaling smell before undergoing a therapy.

Automobile manufacturers could develop air conditioners with a preset mechanism to discharge aromas to keep the drivers alert while driving.

There are two simple tests to train your nose to learn and memorise the various smells. Test I would tell you how good your sense of smell is and Test II would tell you which aroma or essential oil you like the best.

Test I: Sniff and tell test

Blind fold your eyes and ask your friend or a family member to bring ten items from your kitchen . Let your partner allow you to sniff the item one by one and then try to recognise them by their aroma without actually seeing them. The items could be freshly cut citrus fruit, freshly crushed herbs, jars containing pickle, sauce etc. Place the items three inches away from the tip of your nose for about 30 seconds. You should guess all the items correctly. If you are successful in guessing a minimum of 5-6 items then it means that your sense of smell is above average. However, one should aim to develop 100% sense of smell.

Test II: The scent family test

Pick nine essential oils viz. three from the floral family, three from spicy family and three from green family. Mix them up and smell them randomly. You can smell them with your eyes closed for better concentration. This test will enable you to find out which aroma category you like the most. Maybe you like the floral smells better than the scent of the oil from the green family.

An aromatherapist should at least stock 30-40 types of oils. It is advisable to go in for the aromas you are naturally attracted to rather than all the essential oils that are available in the market.

The Best essential oils

Almost all the useful oils mix well with many other oils. Their combination have the broadest range of therapeutic uses, in addition to the most pleasant fragrance.

One can start by using a mixture of two or three or all of the following essential oils.

To begin use Lavender, Neroli, Peppermint, Sandalwood, Rose and one can add to them Eucalyptus, Geranium, Lemon, Patchouli, Chamomile, Ylang Ylang.

The five fragrance categories are:

Green

Basil	Chamomile
Clarysage	Eucalyptus

Galbanum
Peppermint
Pine
Rosemary
Thyme

Floral

Lavender
Geranium
Rose
Neroli
Ylang Ylang

Citrus

Lemon
Lemongrass
Orange
Bergamot
Petitgrain

Woody

Cedarwood
Frankincense
Patchouli
Sandalwood

Spicy

Camphor
Fennel
Ginger
Juniper

Marjoram
Tarragon
Tea-tree

Mixing of aroma oils

Basil can be mixed with

Bergamot
Cypress
Eucalyptus
Frankincense
Geranium
Ginger
Juniper
Lavender
Lemon
Lemongrass
Tea-tree
Peppermint
Petitgrain
Pine
Rosemary
Clarysage
Tarragon
Thyme
Ylang Ylang

Bergamot can be mixed with

Basil
Cedarwood
Cypress
Fennel

Chamomile
Ginger
Juniper
Lavender
Lemon
Lemongrass
Marjoram
Neroli
Orange
Patchouli
Peppermint
Geranium
Petitgrain
Pine
Rose
Rosemary
Clarysage
Sandalwood
Tea-tree
Thyme
Ylang Ylang

Camphor can be mixed with

Cedarwood
Cypress
Frankincense
Ginger
Peppermint
Pine
Rosemary
Tarragon
Tea-tree

Cedarwood can be mixed with

Bergamot
Camphor
Chamomile
Cypress
Eucalyptus
Fennel
Frankincense
Geranium
Juniper
Lavender
Lemon
Neroli
Orange
Peppermint
Pine
Rosemary
Clarysage

Cypress can be mixed with

Basil
Bergamot
Camphor
Cedarwood
Chamomile
Eucalyptus
Fennel
Frankincense
Geranium
Juniper
Lavender
Lemon
Patchouli
Pine

Rose	Clarysage
Rosemary	Sandalwood

Eucalyptus can be mixed with

Basil	Lemon
Cedarwood	Marjoram
Chamomile	Peppermint
Cypress	Peppermint
Fennel	Pine
Frankincense	Rosemary
Geranium	Clarysage
Ginger	Sandalwood
Juniper	Tea-tree
Lavender	Thyme

Fennel can be mixed with

Bergamot	Eucalyptus
Cedarwood	Frankincense
Chamomile	Geranium
Cypress	Ginger

Juniper
Lavender
Lemon
Peppermint
Rose
Rosemary
Sandalwood

Frankincense can be mixed with

Basil
Camphor
Cedarwood
Chamomile
Cypress
Eucalyptus
Frankincense
Fennel
Geranium
Ginger
Juniper
Lavender
Lemon
Neroli
Patchouli
Pine
Rose
Rosemary

Geranium can be mixed with

Basil
Bergamot
Cedarwood
Chamomile
Cypress
Eucalyptus

Frankincense
Fennel
Juniper
Lavender
Lemon
Lemongrass
Clarysage
Sandalwood
Ylang Ylang

Ginger can be mixed with

Basil
Bergamot
Camphor
Eucalyptus
Frankincense
Fennel
Neroli
Orange
Patchouli
Rose
Rosemary
Clarysage
Sandalwood
Ylang Ylang

Juniper can be mixed with

Basil
Bergamot
Cedarwood
Chamomile
Cypress
Eucalyptus
Fennel
Frankincense

Geranium
Lavender
Lemon
Neroli
Peppermint
Petitgrain
Rose
Rosemary
Clarysage
Sandalwood
Ylang Ylang

Lavender can be mixed with

Basil
Bergamot
Cedarwood
Chamomile
Cypress
Eucalyptus
Fennel
Frankincense
Geranium
Juniper
Lemon
Lemongrass
Marjoram
Peppermint
Petitgrain
Pine
Rosemary
Clarysage
Sandalwood
Tarragon
Tea-tree
Thyme

Lemon can be mixed with

Basil
Bergamot
Cedarwood
Chamomile
Cypress
Eucalyptus
Fennel
Frankincense
Geranium
Lavender
Marjoram
Neroli
Orange
Petitgrain
Pine
Patchouli
Rose
Rosemary
Sandalwood
Tea-tree
Ylang Ylang

Marjoram can be mixed with

Basil
Bergamot
Chamomile
Eucalyptus
Geranium
Ginger
Juniper
Lavender
Lemon
Lemongrass
Neroli
Rose

Rosemary
Clarysage
Sandalwood
Ylang Ylang

Neroli can be mixed with

Bergamot
Cedarwood
Chamomile
Geranium
Ginger
Juniper
Lavender
Lemon
Marjoram
Orange
Patchouli
Rose
Rosemary
Sandalwood
Ylang Ylang

Orange can be mixed with

Bergamot
Cedarwood
Frankincense
Geranium
Ginger
Lavender
Lemon
Lemongrass
Neroli
Patchouli
Petitgrain
Pine

Rosemary
Clarysage
Sandalwood

Patchouli can be mixed with

Bergamot
Chamomile
Cypress
Frankincense
Ginger
Lavender
Lemon
Marjoram
Orange
Peppermint
Pine
Rose
Clarysage
Sandalwood
Ylang Ylang

Peppermint can mixed with

Basil
Bergamot
Camphor
Cedarwood
Eucalyptus
Fennel
Juniper
Lemon
Lavender
Patchouli

Rose
Rosemary
Clarysage
Sandalwood

Petitgrain can be mixed with

Basil
Bergamot
Lavender
Lemon
Orange
Rosemary
Sandalwood
Ylang Ylang

Pine can be mixed with

Basil
Camphor
Cedarwood
Chamomile
Cypress
Eucalyptus
Frankincense
Lavender
Lemon
Orange
Patchouli
Rosemary
Tea-tree

Rose can be mixed with

Bergamot
Chamomile
Cypress
Frankincense

Fennel
Geranium
Ginger
Juniper
Lavender
Lemon
Marjoram
Neroli
Patchouli
Peppermint
Clarysage
Sandalwood
Thyme

Rosemary can be mixed with

Basil
Bergamot
Cedarwood
Camphor
Chamomile
Cypress
Eucalyptus
Fennel
Frankincense
Geranium
Juniper
Lavender
Lemon
Lemongrass
Marjoram
Neroli
Orange
Peppermint
Pine
Patchouli
Sandalwood
Thyme

Clary Sage can be mixed with

Basil	Lemon
Bergamot	Lemongrass
Cedarwood	Marjoram
Cypress	Orange
Eucalyptus	Patchouli
Frankincense	Peppermint
Geranium	Rose
Ginger	Sandalwood
Juniper	Ylang Ylang
Lavender	

Sandalwood can be mixed with

Bergamot	Ginger
Cypress	Juniper
Chamomile	Lavender
Eucalyptus	Lavender
Frankincense	Marjoram
Fennel	Neroli
Geranium	Orange

Patchouli	Clarysage
Peppermint	Clarysage
Rose	Ylang Ylang
Rosemary	

Tea-tree can be mixed with

Bergamot	Ginger
Chamomile	Juniper
Cypress	Lavender
Eucalyptus	Lemon
Frankincense	Pine
Fennel	Sandalwood
Geranium	

Tarragon can be mixed with

Basil	Cedarwood
Camphor	Lemongrass

Thyme can be mixed with

Basil	Chamomile
Bergamot	Eucalyptus

Lavender	Rosemary
Lemon	Clarysage

Ylang Ylang can be mixed with

Basil	Neroli
Bergamot	Patchouli
Frankincense	Petitgrain
Geranium	Pine
Ginger	Rose
Juniper	Clarysage
Lavender	Sandalwood
Lemon	Thyme
Marjoram	

Aroma oils for common problems

Aroma oils are either relaxing, calming, stimulating or have therapeutic qualities. While using the essential oils care should be taken to dilute the oils before application.

Acne

Oils: Bergamot, Cedarwood, Geranium, Lavender, Juniper, Sandalwood, Lemon, Tea-tree, Chamomile, Petitgrain, Patchouli and Lemongrass.

Anxiety and Stress

Oils: Lavender, Neroli, Patchouli, Sandalwood, Bergamot, Frankincense, Clarysage and Ylang Ylang.

Athlete's Foot
Oils: Lavender, Tea-tree, Geranium and Lemongrass.

Arthritis
Oils: Eucalyptus, Ginger, Juniper, Pine, Peppermint, Cypress, Rosemary and Lemon.

Backache
Oils: Camphor, Eucalyptus, Pine, Juniper, Petitgrain, Rosemary, Lavender, Clarysage and Thyme.

Bites and stings
Oils: Basil, Chamomile, Lavender, Peppermint and Tea-tree.

Breathing problems
Oils: Cedarwood, Eucalyptus, Peppermint, Pine, Rosemary, Sandalwood and Tea-tree.

Bunion

Bunion is a painful inflammation of the joint between the big toe and the foot which is sometimes caused due to ill-fitting shoes

Oils: Cypress, Lemon and Peppermint.

Bruises

Oils: Camphor, Clarysage, Cypress, Geranium and Lavender.

Burns

Oils: Chamomile, Geranium, Lavender, Rose and Tea-tree.

Cellulite

Cellulite (common in women) is a lumpy, dimpled, orange-peel like appearance on thighs, bottom and back of arms. It is usually caused due to accumulation of fluid and toxins in the tissues because of lack of proper circulation and hormonal fluctuations. Regular massage with aroma oils can help to smoothen the lumps.

Oils: Cedarwood, Clarysage, Cypress, Geranium, Fennel, Juniper, Lemon, Lavender and Patchouli.

Chickenpox

Oils: Bergamot, Chamomile, Eucalyptus, Lavender and Tea-tree.

Chilblains

Chilblains is seen as discoloured, swollen veins on the fingers, toes and the back of legs after exposure to extremely cold weather.

Oils: Cypress, Eucalyptus, Ginger, Juniper, Lemon, Lemongrass, Marjoram, Rosemary and Tea-tree.

Circulation (poor)

Oils: Basil, Cypress, Cedarwood, Clarysage, Ginger, Juniper, Lemon, Lemongrass, Lavender, Peppermint, Pine, Rosemary and Ylang Ylang.

Cold

Oils: Camphor, Eucalyptus, Lavender, Lemon, Marjoram, Peppermint, Pine, Tea-tree and Thyme.

Cough

Oils: Cedarwood, Cypress, Eucalyptus, Frankincense, Ginger, Lemon, Pine, Peppermint, Rosemary, Sandalwood and Thyme.

Cramps
Oils: Chamomile, Eucalyptus, Fennel, Juniper, Lemon, Lavender, Marjoram, Neroli, Tarragon and Ylang Ylang.

Cuts and Abrasions
Oils: Bergamot, Chamomile, Geranium, Lavender and Tea-tree.

Dandruff
Oils: Cedarwood, Geranium, Juniper, Lemon, Lavender, Rosemary, Sandalwood and Tea-tree.

Depression
Oils: Bergamot, Geranium, Clarysage, Sandalwood, Rose, Frankincense, Neroli and Lavender, Ylang Ylang.

Dermatitis, Psoriasis, Eczema

Oils: Bergamot, Cedarwood, Chamomile, Geranium, Lavender, Sandalwood and Cypress.

Fatigue

Oils: Basil, Bergamot, Geranium, Frankincense, Eucalyptus, Lavender, Lemon, Peppermint, Clarysage, Thyme, Ginger, Patchouli, Fennel and Orange.

Fluid Retention

Oils: Geranium, Fennel, Patchouli, Cypress, Juniper and Rosemary.

Fungal Infection

Oils: Lavender, Tea-tree, Geranium, Lemongrass, Juniper and Sandalwood.

Hair Loss

Oils: Rosemary, Lavender, Clarysage, Cedarwood and Ylang Ylang.

Hair (oily)

Oils: Rosemary, Lavender, Cypress, Geranium, Lemon and Tea-tree.

Hair (dry)

Oils: Chamomile for blonde hair, Rosemary, Lavender for red, brown hair and Tea-tree for dandruff.

Hangover

Oils: Geranium, Lavender, Rose, Neroli, Lemon and Peppermint.

Headache

Oils: Eucalyptus, Frankincense, Chamomile, Peppermint, Clarysage, Lavender, Rose, Lemongrass and

Thyme.

Herpes

Oils: Bergamot, Chamomile, Eucalyptus, Lavender, Lemon, Patchouli and Tea-tree.

Household Cleansers

Oils: Geranium, Lavender Chamomile, Eucalyptus, Lemon, Tea-tree, Bergamot, Lemongrass, Thyme, Peppermint and Pine.

Indigestion

Oils: Fennel, Lavender, Peppermint, Marjoram and Tarragon.

Influenza

Oils: Eucalyptus, Peppermint, Pine, Tea-tree, Thyme, Marjoram, Orange and Rosemary.

Insomnia

Oils: Geranium, Basil, Lavender, Chamomile, Rose, Cypress, Petitgrain, Neroli, Marjoram, Sandalwood and Ylang Ylang

Insect Repellents

Oils: Camphor, Lemongrass, Basil, Tea-tree and Thyme.

Measles

Oils: Bergamot, Eucalyptus, Chamomile, Lavender and Tea-tree.

Menopause

Oils: Chamomile, Rose, Lavender, Cypress, Geranium, Clarysage, Peppermint and Ylang Ylang.

Nausea

Oils: Ginger, Lemon and Peppermint.

Perspiration or Excess Sweating

Oils: Bergamot, Lemongrass, Lavender and Thyme.

Premenstrual tension

Oils: Bergamot, Clarysage, Cypress, Chamomile, Fennel, Geranium, Juniper, Lavender, Peppermint, Rose, Sandalwood and Tarragon.

Rheumatism

Oils: Cypress, Chamomile, Eucalyptus, Ginger, Juniper, Lavender, Lemon, Marjoram and Rosemary.

Sexual Problems

Oils: Clarysage, Ginger, Geranium, Neroli, Patchouli, Rose, Sandalwood and Ylang Ylang.

Skin(Mature)

Oils: Chamomile, Frankincense, Geranium, Lavender, Neroli, Orange, Rosemary, Rose and Ylang Ylang.

Skin(Thread Vein)

Oils: Chamomile, Cypress, Geranium, Orange and Lemon.

Skin(Dry and Sensitive)

Oils: Chamomile, Geranium, Lavender, Neroli, Patchouli, Rose, Sandalwood and Tea-tree.

Skin(Oily and Blemished)

Oils: Bergamot, Chamomile, Geranium, Lavender, Neroli, Cedarwood, Juniper, Lemongrass,

Petitgrain, Patchouli, Lemon and Thyme.

Stress

Oils: Basil, Bergamot, Lavender, Neroli Chamomile, Geranium, Frankincense, Clarysage, Patchouli, Marjoram, Sandalwood and Ylang Ylang.

Sunburn

Oils: Chamomile, Geranium, Lavender and Rose.

Travel Sickness

Oils: Bergamot, Ginger, Lemon and Peppermint.

Specific Features of Aroma oils

Analgesic (To reduce pain)
Oils: Bergamot, Chamomile, Lavender, Marjoram and Rosemary.

Antidepressant (To lift the mood)
Oils: Bergamot, Clarysage, Chamomile, Geranium, Lavender, Neroli, Petitgrain, Rose, Orange, Sandalwood and Ylang Ylang.

Anaphrodisiac (To decrease sexual Response)
Oil: Marjoram.

Anti-Inflammatory (To reduce inflammation)
Oil: Bergamot, Chamomile and Lavender.

Antiseptic (To fight bacteria locally)
Oil: Bergamot, Eucalyptus, Lavender, Juniper, Rosemary, Tea-tree and Sandalwood.

Antiviral
Oils: Tea-tree and Lavender.

Astringent
Oils: Cypress, Cedarwood, Juniper, Frankincense, Sandalwood and Rose.

Aphrodisiac (Enhance Sexuality)
Oils: Rose, Neroli, Clarysage, Sandalwood and Ylang Ylang.

Bactericide (Kills bacteria)
Oils: Bergamot, Eucalyptus, Lavender, Juniper, Rosemary and Neroli.

Cephalic (Clears the mind, stimulates mental activity)
Oils: Basil and Rosemary.

Chalagogue (To stimulate the flow of bile)
Oils: Chamomile, Lavender, Peppermint and Rosemary.

Cytophylactic (Regenerates cell)
Oils: Frankincense, Tea-tree, Lavender, Neroli and Palmarosa.

Deodarant (Reduces odour)
Oils: Clarysage, Lavender, Neroli, Petitgrain, Eucalyptus, Lavender and Cypress.

Detoxifying (Cleanses the body of impurities)
Oils: Fennel, Juniper and Rose.

Diuretic (To increase production of urine)
Oils: Cypress, Cedarwood, Chamomile, Frankincense, Fennel, Geranium, Juniper, Rosemary and Sandalwood.

Emmenagogue (To encourage menstruation)
Oils: Basil, Clarysage, Chamomile, Juniper, Lavender, Marjoram, Rose and Rosemary.

Expectorant (To expel phlegm)
Oils: Bergamot, Eucalyptus, Marjoram and Sandalwood.

Febrifuge (To reduce fever)
Oils: Bergamot, Chamomile, Eucalyptus, Tea-tree and Peppermint.

Fungicidal (To arrest growth of yeasts, moulds)
Oils: Lavender and Tea-tree.

Hepatic (To strengthen liver)
Oils: Chamomile, Lemon, Cypress, Rosemary, Tea-tree and Lavender.

Hypertensive (To raise blood pressure)
Oils: Rosemary and Clarysage.

Hypnotic (To induce alpha state)
Oils: Chamomile, Lavender, Neroli, Marjoram and Ylang Ylang.

Hypotensive (To lower blood pressure)
Oils: Marjoram, Lavender and Ylang Ylang.

Immuno-Stimulant (To strengthen the body's defensive reaction to infection)
Oils: Lavender and Tea-tree

Nervine (To strengthen the nervous system)
Oils: Chamomile, Lavender, Marjoram and Rosemary.

Sedative (To calm the nervous system)
Oils: Bergamot, Clarysage, Juniper, Frankincense, Lavender, Marjoram, Rose, Neroli and Sandalwood.

Stimulant (Enhances the body activity)
Oils: Black Pepper, Eucalyptus, Geranium, Rosemary and Peppermint.

Tonic (To strengthen the body generally)

Oils: Black Pepper, Basil, Chamomile, Geranium, Frankincense, Lavender, Juniper, Marjoram, Rose, Neroli and Tea-tree.

Oils to be used in moderation

Basil	Clarysage
Camphor	Tarragon
Fennel	Thyme
Ginger	

Oils that are photo-toxic or photosensitive

Photo-toxic or photosensitivity is a reaction to essential oils causing redness, increased pigmentation and problems of the skin when in contact with the sunlight or excessive light. There is a possibility that the oils that cause photosensitivity can increase the likelihood of damage to the skin.

Bergamot	Neroli
Cedarwood	Orange(sweet and bitter)
Clarysage	Patchouli
Ginger	
Lemon	

Oils to be avoided in Pregnancy

Rosemary	Clarysage
Basil	Cedarwood
Fennel	Juniper
Thyme	Tarragon
Marjoram	

Oils that can cause skin irritation

Basil	Lavender
Bergamot	Lemon
Black pepper	Lemongrass

Camphor
Cedarwood
Chamomile
Clove bud
Eucalyptus
Geranium
Ginger
Juniper
Neroli
Peppermint
Pine
Sandalwood
Tea-tree
Thyme
Vetiver
Ylang Ylang

Avoid using the essential oils undiluted and insist on a skin patch test before using the aroma oils extensively on a regular basis.

Oils to be avoided while on Homeopathic medicines

The oils given below, when used while under Homeopathic medicine could neutralise the benefits of the Homeopathic remedies therefore they should be avoided.

Black Pepper	Eucalyptus
Camphor	Peppermint
Clove bud	Rosemary

Oils to be avoided when driving(long distance).

The following oils should be avoided when driving because these can cause drowsiness when one has to be alert.

Chamomile	Petitgrain
Geranium	Rose
Lavender	Sandalwood
Marjoram	Vetiver
Neroli	Ylang Ylang

Oils that can be contra-indicators during certain illness

Condition		*Contra-indicator oil*
Asthma	:	Marjoram, Camphor, Rosemary.

Anorexia	:	Patchouli.
Cancer	:	Basil, Fennel.
Epilepsy	:	Clarysage, Fennel, Eucalyptus, Lavender, Rosemary.
Hypertension	:	Rosemary, Thyme.
Hypotension	:	Marjoram, Clarysage.
Liver disease	:	Clove bud, Thyme, Vetiver.
Ulcers of the stomach and intestine	:	Cinnamon.

Carrier Oils

Carrier oils or base oils are vegetable, nut or seed oils. Many of these carrier oils also have therapeutic properties. Vegetable oils are extracted from the seeds of the plants. Vegetable oils contain a good amount of proteins, nutrients and energy. They enable the body to produce heat and lubrication.

The essential oils are very highly concentrated and cannot be used directly on the skin. The essential oils are hence diluted with a base or carrier oil so that they can be massaged or rubbed into the skin in the correct proportion.

Almond Oil (Sweet)

Colour	:	very pale yellow.
Extracted	:	from the kernel.
Contains	:	glycosides, minerals, vitamins and proteins.
Uses	:	good for skin, helps relieve itching, soreness, dryness and inflammation.
Base oil	:	can be used as a base without dilution.

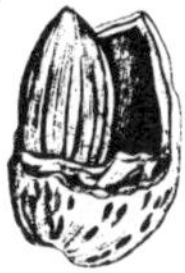

Apricot kernel oil

Colour	:	pale yellow.
Extracted	:	from the kernel.
Contains	:	minerals, vitamins.
Uses	:	all types of skin particularly for prematured aged,

		sensitive, inflammed and dry skin.
Base oil	:	can be used as a base without dilution.

Avocado pear oil

Colour	:	dark green.
Extracted	:	from the fruit.
Contains	:	vitamins, proteins, lecithin and fatty acids.
Uses	:	all types of skin especially dry and dehydrated skin, eczema.
Base oil	:	to be used as an addition to a base oil in 10% dilution.

Carrot oil

Colour	:	Orange.
Contains	:	vitamins, minerals, and beta-carotene.
Uses	:	premature aging, itching, dryness, psoriasis and eczema. Very rejuvenating by itself and reduces scarring.
Base oil	:	to be used as an addition to a base oil in 10% dilution. Do not use undiluted directly on the skin.

Corn oil

Colour	:	pale yellow.
Contains	:	vitamins, minerals and protein.

Uses	:	Soothing for all types of skin.
Base oil	:	can be used as base oil.

Evening Primrose

Colour	:	pale yellow.
Contains	:	gamma linolenic acid, vitamins and minerals.
Uses	:	during Pre menstrual tension, multiple sclerosis, menopause related tensions heart diseases. Excellent while treating eczema and psoriasis. Helps prevent premature aging of skin.

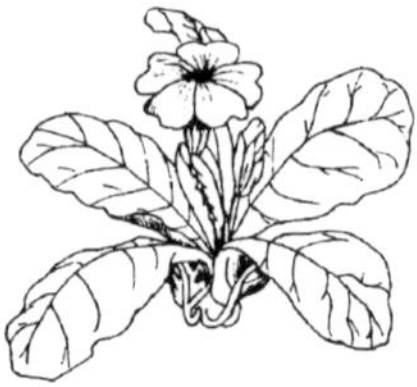

Base oil	:	use in 10% dilution.

Grapeseed oil

Colour	:	nearly colourless or pale green.
Contains	:	vitamins, minerals and protein.
Uses	:	for all types of skin.
Base oil	:	can be used as base oil without dilution.

Hazelnut oil

Colour	:	yellow.
Extracted	:	from the kernel.
Contains	:	vitamins, minerals and protein.
Uses	:	for all types of skin. It has a slight astringent action.
Base oil	:	use with 10% dilution.

Jojoba oil

Colour	:	yellow.
Extracted	:	from the bean.
Contains	:	minerals, protein, a waxy substance similar to collagen.
Uses	:	for inflammed skins, psoriasis, eczema, acne, hair care. It can be used on all types of skin as it is a very penetrative oil.
Base oil	:	can be used as base oil without dilution.

Olive oil

Colour	:	green.
Contains	:	vitamins, minerals, protein.

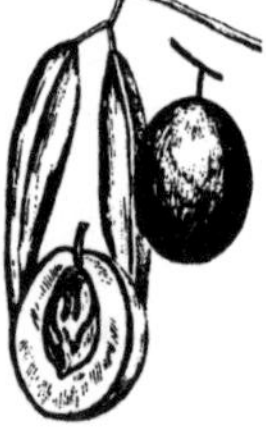

Uses	:	rheumatism, hair care, cosmetics. It is a very soothing oil.
Base oil	:	use in 10% dilution.

Peanut oil

Colour	:	pale yellow.
Contains	:	vitamins, minerals and protein.
Uses	:	for all types of skin.
Base oil	:	can be used as base oil without dilution.

Safflower oil

Colour	:	pale yellow.
Contains	:	vitamins, minerals and protein.
Uses	:	for all types of skin.
Base oil	:	can be used as base oil without dilution.

Sesame oil

Colour	:	dark yellow.
Contains	:	vitamins, minerals, protein, lecithin and amino acids.
Uses	:	rheumatism, arthritis, psoriasis, eczema. Useful for all skin types.
Base oil	:	use in 10% dilution.

Soya bean oil

Colour	:	pale yellow.
Contains	:	vitamins, minerals and protein.
Uses	:	for all types of skin.
Base oil	:	can be used as base oil without dilution.

Sunflower oil

Colour	:	pale yellow.

Contains	:	vitamins and minerals.
Uses	:	for all types of skin.
Base oil	:	can be used as base oil without dilution.

Equipment required for mixing oils

After studying the feature, properties or category, select the essential oils you wish to mix and use. It is preferable not to mix more than three oils at a time for use. Also select the oils belonging to the same category. For example if you want to use more than one oil select them all from either floral, spicy, citrus, green or woody. Hence you could try out a mixture of perhaps lavender, rose and ylang ylang as all these belong to the floral family.

Once you have selected the oils you want to mix and use, try the combination in a smaller quantity before you mix a large quantity so as to not waste the oils. Cut long strips of blotting paper, drop a drop each of the selected oils in case you wish to use equal amount of all the oils selected. In case you have decided to use any one or two of the selected oil more than the other, add two drops of those. Now hold the strip and move the oily tip of the blotting paper backward and forward under your nose as you inhale the aroma. Allow your sense of smell to be the judge and guide you in selecting the combinations.

Since aromatherapy is very personal you should get the other person to do a similar test before mixing a combination because it is not necessary that the mixture selected by you and liked by you should necessarily be liked by others too.

Equipment

- A 10 ml dark coloured glass bottles with stoppered caps for storing pure essential oils.
- Four eye-droppers or pipettes. You could use one only if you thoroughly wash it every time after every use.
- A small funnel for pouring carrier oils into bottles.
- A large, dark coloured glass, stoppered bottles for storing the combinations of oils or a ceramic bowl for immediate use. Please do not use metal containers or bowls.
- Strips of blotting paper.

How to select essential oils

The Best Aroma Oils:

Clary Sage	Peppermint
Eucalyptus	Petitgrain
Geranium	Rosemary
Lavender	Tea Tree
Lemon	Ylang Ylang

Male Favourites:

Basil	Lemon
Bergamot	Patchouli
Eucalyptus	Pine
Frankincense	Sandalwood
Lavender	

Female Favourites:

Bergamot	Lavender
Geranium	Neroli

Patchouli
Peppermint
Rose
Clarysage
Ylang Ylang

Caution to be exercised while using aroma oils

Skin Patch Test

To test aroma oil blended with carrier or base oils

- Wash and dry the forearm thoroughly.
- Apply just a few drops of the blended aroma oil to moisten the area.
- Cover the area with a sterile gauze.
- Let it remain for 24 hours.
- If there is irritation then wash immediately.
- In case of irritation, you should not use this oil.

To test essential oil in its pure state

- Wash and dry the forearm thoroughly with an unscented vegetable soap.
- Apply one drop of the aroma oil to the crook of the arm.
- Bend the arm so that it touches the shoulder for five minutes.
- Open and close once more.

If any irritation occurs wash immediately with water and soap or wipe carefully with a cotton ball soaked in milk and vegetable oil.

In case accidental poisoning occurs follow the following :

Aroma oils being potent, safety precautions need to be followed with utmost care. Do not allow children to play with these oils and always store them away from the reach of children and other non-qualified users of essential oils.

In eyes

In case essential oil comes in contact with the eyes, do not rinse with water. But instead wipe the eye with a ball of cotton soaked in milk or vegetable oil. If irritation still persists wash the eyes with water poured from a jug, from a height of 3-5 inches for 15 minutes. Consult a doctor. It always helps to wash the eyes for 10 to 15 minutes than splashing it with running water.

Toxic effects

Toxic effects can happen when the oil is not evenly spread out on the area and remains concentrated in one area in a large quantity. Even daily exposure to the same oil on a regular basis for a prolonged period can lead to toxicity. Symptoms that would follow a toxic reaction are fatigue, headaches, liver pain, liver enlargement, coughing and urine disturbances. This make it mandatory for the therapists using essential oils to work in a well ventilated room and wash their hands thoroughly after handling the oils.

Allergic effects

An allergic reaction to aroma oil would result in nausea, dizziness, sweating, stomach pain, mucous membrane, irritation and palpitation. These allergic reactions are temporary and would cease to exist as soon as the use of the essential oils is stopped.

The following precautions needs to be followed while dealing with essential oils having toxic rating

The toxicity of the essential oils depends on the level of toxicity and concentration of the chemical compounds. All aroma oils need to be used as per instructions only and more so when handling those essential oils under toxic listing. Normally a toxic reaction occurs when the essential oil is used in excess or incorrectly. It is safer to use the aroma oils under proper guidance and instructions.

- Do not exceed the recommended dosage.

- If you feel uncomfortable even while using the recommended dosage reduce the dosage to half.
- Follow the skin patch test carefully.
- Avoid usage for a long period. The maximum administration time should not exceed two -four weeks. Leave a gap of 30 days before beginning to use again.
- Avoid use during pregnancy.
- Do not use if you are a nursing mother.
- Do not administer on infants, small children , frail or elderly people who have less resistance.

Different ways of using Essential oils

Method and Usage

Rub oil : 8-10 drops of essential oil in 10ml base oil. Use only 4-6 drops once a day preferably at night

Baths : 6-8 drops in a tub, 2-3 drops in a bucket once a day

Shower : 10-12 drops in 10 ml base oil once a day. Wash as usual. Add oil on your face towel, cloth or sponge or even your hands and rub briskly all over the body as you stand under the running shower. Breathe deeply

	to benefit from the aromatic vapour.
Massage oil	: 8-10 drops of essential oil for every 30 ml of vegetable base oil once a day
Diffuser	: 1-6 drops
Inhalation	: 2-3 drops once a day
Tissue	: 1-2 drops on a tissue. Sniff when required. Keep the tissue under the pillow during the night
Cotton balls	: 2-3 drops of essential oil on a piece of cotton and left for 10-15 minutes to dry. This piece of cotton can be kept in the cupboard, car, shoe rack, lockers etc.

Water bowls	: 1-9 drops of aroma oil to be added to bowl of boiling water. Keep in the room and close the windows, door and allow the aroma to spread in the room. This can also be used in the work places.
Room sprays	: 4-6 drops can be added to 30 ml of water in a spray bottle. Shake well and spray the mixture in the air. Avoid spraying directly on delicate machines. Ideal for home and office use.

Careful handling of the essential oils

- Essential oils are not recommended for internal consumption
- Certain oils are to be avoided during early pregnancy as they can induce menstruation and some even have diuretic properties which can deplete the fluid in the foetal sack. These oils include basil, clarysage, rose-mary, juniper, marjoram, clove bud, fennel, cypress, peppermint, cedarwood. However this caution does not apply to oils used in vaporisers.

- Avoid exposure to sun for at least four hours after using essential oils as some oils can make the skin photosensitive to ultraviolet rays from the sun. Bergamot, lemon, orange, petitgrain are some such oils that can cause photo-sensitivity.
- People suffering from high blood pressure, epilepsy, neural disorders or kidney disease should avoid some oils viz. Black pepper, rosemary, cypress, juniper.
- Aroma oils are not a substitute for any drugs being taken under the advice of a qualified physician for serious ailments. It is always advisable to consult a qualified therapist before considering the

use of essential oils particularly when suffering from serious ailments.

- Use the oils in recommended dosage. Usage in excess can lead to opposite effect to that which you are trying to achieve and there are chances of building up of the toxicity within the body. Ylang ylang, marjoram, clarysage need to be used with utmost precaution.
- Essential oils should always be used diluted unless recommended otherwise.
- Keep out of reach of children
- Store the oils only in dark glass containers. The colour of the bottle should preferably be amber rather than cobalt blue.

Only blended oils should be stored in cobalt blue bottles.

- Store in a cool, dark place away from sunlight to prolong the life of the aroma oils and also to preserve the therapeutic powers of the essential oils.
- Avoid using essential oils near the eyes or other sensitive areas.
- Avoid contact with plastic, varnished or painted surfaces.
- When blending essential oils use a stainless steel, glass or ceramic container and not plastic.
- Do not use essential oils on newborn. Use only one drop of lavender in the bath until the age of four months. For the use of essential oils on children up to the age of 12 years, all the

essential oil dosage given to an adult must be divided into 4 portion.

- What suits one may not necessarily suit another person.
- Avoid certain aroma oils under the influence of alcohol. Oils viz. clarysage, marjoram, ylang ylang should particularly be avoided in case alcohol has been taken.
- Some oils may irritate the skin. Always do a skin patch test before applying the oils to larger area.
- If you are not sure of a particular blend, it is always better to take advise from a professional aromatherapist.

How aroma oils are made

- Distillation

Water distillation for dried material that will not get damaged by boiling. This method is also used for powdered materials and flowers like rose and orange flowers

Water and Steam distillation for dried and fresh material that would get damaged by boiling. In this method they are supported on a perforated grid and steam is passed through them like cinnamon and clove.

Direct steam distillation for fresh plant material having a high boiling point, steam is passed at a high temperature (seeds, roots, wood). Also applicable for fresh plant material like peppermint.

- *Cold pressing or expression* is mainly for citrus oils like lemon and orange. The fruit is rolled over sharp projections that puncture the oil glands. Fruit is then pressed to remove the oil and then washed off with a fine spray of water. Rotating the mixture at a very high speed separates oil and water. The fruit can also first be separated from the peel and then cold pressed like bergamot.

- *Carbon dioxide extraction* – Liquid co_2 is used as a solvent to extract essential oils. Liquefied under pressure, it acts as a solvent, reverting back to gaseous nature when pressure is reduced leaving no trace of solvent.

• *Solvent extraction* – Volatile solvents like petroleum, ether, benzene or hexane are mixed into petals till the essential oil is completely dissolved. Filtration is followed by reduced pressure and evaporation of the solvent to give concrete products which contains insoluble vegetation wax or pigments. On continuing the process with solvents and freezing it finally separates the waxes and gives the final product which is called absolute.

Aroma oil and beauty care

Suggested blends for skin types

Normal skin	:	Lavender, Geranium, Rosemary, Cedarwood, Orange.
Dry skin	:	Lavender, Geranium, Cedarwood, Patchouli, Frankincense, Sandalwood, Ylang Ylang.
Oily skin	:	Cedarwood, Lavender, Rosemary, Frankincense, Orange, Cypress, Bergamot, Juniper, Lemongrass, Clarysage, Lemon.

Mature skin	:	Frankincense, Sandalwood, Ylang Ylang, Patchouli, Cypress, Lavender, Geranium.
Blemished skin	:	Lavender, Geranium, Rosemary, Lemon, Tea-tree.
Sensitive skin	:	Lavender, Sandalwood, Cedarwood.

Moisturisers

Add the following blends to 50 ml of unscented moisturiser base

Day Cream (dry skin)

2 drop of Wheat Germ
4 drops of Lavender
2 drops of Ylang Ylang
4 drops of Frankincense

Night cream (Dry skin)
1 ml Jojoba
6 drops of Geranium
4 drops of Sandalwood
2 drops of Frankincense

Pimple ointment
8 drops of Lavender
1 drop of Peppermint
4 drops of Tea tree

Day Cream(Oily skin)
2 drops of Wheat Germ
2 drops of Lemon
3 drops of Lavender
2 drops of Cypress
2 drops of Juniper

Hair care

Suggested oils for hair types

Dry hair	:	Rosemary, Sandalwood, Ylang Ylang, Lavender, Geranium, Frankincense, Patchouli.
Oily hair	:	Basil, Eucalyptus, Cedarwood, Lemongrass, Cypress, Rosemary, Bergamot, Juniper.
Normal hair	:	Geranium, Lemon, Lemongrass, Clary-sage, Cedarwood, Rosemary.

Dandruff	:	Cedarwood, Eucalyptus, Clarysage, Patchouli, Rosemary, Tea tree, Lavender.
Brittled or Damaged	:	Sandalwood, Geranium, Frankincense, Lavender, Patchouli.

A special scalp treatment for brittle or damaged hair:

Take 10 ml Jojoba

5 drops of dry hair type combination

Method: Warm the blends in a dish. Massage the mixture into the scalp. Saturate some cotton wool and rub through to the ends of the hair. Wrap a hot towel around your head. Leave for 15 minutes and then shampoo.

Treat your feet

Tired feet :

2 drops of Orange
3 drops of Rosemary
3 drops of Lavender

Smelly feet :

3 drops of Cypress
3 drops of Lemongrass
2 drops of Tea tree

Swollen feet :

3 drops of Juniper
3 drops of Lavender
2 drops of Peppermint

Feet Energiser :

3 drops of Bergamot
3 drops of Clarysage
2 drops of Juniper

With the above combination you can enjoy a 15-minute aromatic foot bath at any time of day. These can also be blended and diluted in 20 ml carrier oils to make a refreshing foot massage.

Treat your Hands

Normal skin :
2 drops of Lavender
2 drops of Geranium
3 drops of Sandalwood

Dry skin :
2 drops of Lavender
2 drops of Frankincense
2 drops of Patchouli

Arthritic hands :
3 drops of Juniper

2 drops or Rosemary
1 drop of Cypress

Add any of the above in 15 ml carrier oil and massage into the hands including the forearm. Before the massage soak hands in warm water in which you have dropped 3 drops of Lavender to soften the skin.

How to use aroma oils

All the above oils are ready to use and are mixed with carefully selected carrier oils. They can be used in two ways.

- Rub on the skin locally as required and allow the oil to be absorbed into the blood stream because the oil molecules are so small that they can be absorbed through the pores of the skin or add the aroma oil to the massage oil to obtain higher benefits for the whole body following this by steam or sauna could be a rejuvenating and refreshing feeling.
- Direct inhalation or steam inhalation; sprinkle one or two drops of the chosen oil on a handkerchief

and inhale the oil while at work or travelling. A couple of drops of relaxing oil on a tissue inside your pillow helps you to sleep peacefully. Steam inhalations with two drops of aroma oil in a bowl of hot water also helps. You can also use it in the bath water (in bathtub about 6-8 drops, in bucket 2-3 drops) wraps, compress, massage, inhalation and diffusers. It is advisable to do a patch test before use of any essential oil. Apply at the back of the elbow or wrist and leave for 24 hour without washing the area. If there is no allergy you can comfortably use the oil. Avoid contact with plastic, varnished or painted surfaces. Avoid sensitive areas and eyes. Wash hands after handling the oil. Do not use while taking homeopathic treatment. Do not use for internal consumption. Do not use for babies. Aroma oils are not a substitute for any drugs that are being taken. They can be a complementary therapy. Pregnant ladies and individuals suffering from blood pressure, heart ailment, epilepsy are requested to consult qualified therapists before using essential oils.